My Health Manager©

By Katrina Mulberry BScN

Published by Manage Me, LMS
(Life Management Systems), Inc.

www.ManageMe.ca
Email: info@ManageMe.ca

Copyright, Canadian Copyright Licensing Agency

Library and Archives Canada Cataloguing in Publication.

Issued also in electronic formats.

ISBN 978-0-9869543-1-3

1.   Self-publishing. i. Title

Disclaimer

THE DOCUMENTS PROVIDED PURSUANT TO THIS PROGRAM ARE FOR INFORMATION PURPOSES ONLY.

This information is intended to provide you with the ability to document your medical and health information for your records and to assist you in making appropriate healthcare decisions. Readers should be aware that this publication does not in any way replace consultation with doctors or other health professionals. Nor is it intended to act as a substitute for any problems that may develop from the use or misuse of the information collected.

INFORMATION PROVIDED IN THIS DOCUMENT IS PROVIDED AS IS WITHOUT WARRANTY OF ANY KIND.

The user assumes the entire risk as to the accuracy and the use of this document.

Welcome to My Health Manager ©

My Health **Manager**© is a detailed journal for you to record your own medical history. It is designed to help you track your own health, identify family health patterns and to help you be proactive with your health care needs.

We, at Manage Me, LMS (Life Management Systems) believe that if one maintains their health records, they'll get better health solutions and results by becoming educated health care consumers who are proactive in managing their own health and wellness. After all, it is *your* health.

My Health Manager:

- Embraces preventative health measures through information management
- Reduces redundant medical tests when 2nd opinions are sought
- Reduces the chance of medical errors occurring such as adverse drug interactions and contradictory treatments
- Prevents the loss of important and sometimes critical documentation due to unforeseen events or negligence
- Helps identify familial health patterns and risks for disease states
- Aids your physician and other health care givers, in making health diagnoses and treatments, especially in new patient-health care giver relationships
- Is an act of self responsibility
- Gives you your medical health information when you need it

With **My Health Manager**© in hand, important medical information is not "lost" in a physician's data system. Easy to read tabs provide quick access to one's personal information, medical diagnoses & treatments, medical details such as allergies, eye care, dental care, hearing tests, prescription medications, non-prescription medications, immunizations, family health patterns, surgeries and much more.

My Health Manager © can also be used as a medical alert system, warning physicians about allergies, possible drug interactions or identifying pre-existing medical conditions and family health risks that greatly influence treatment choices.

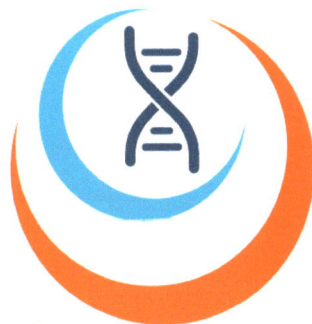

ISBN 978-0-9869543-1-3

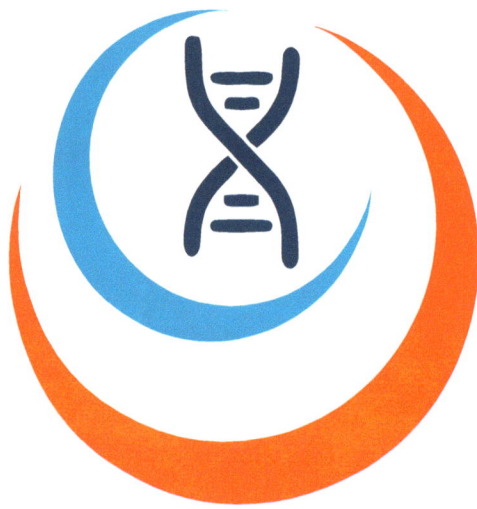

CONTENTS

Personal Information

Last Name		**Date & Place of Birth**	
First Name+ Initial		**Allergies**	
Personal Health Number		**Emergency Conditions**	
Telephone Number		**Blood Type**	
Address		**Organ Donor**	
Emergency Contact Info		**Next of Kin + Contact Info**	

MANAGE ME™
Life Management Services

Personal Information

Sex (M/F)		**Occupation**	
Ethnicity		**Extended Health Care Benefits**	
My Photo Upload		**Circle other Chiro/Physio/ Acupuncture/ Psychiatry/ Dietician/others**	
Eye Colour		**Support Groups**	
Skin Tone		**Research**	
Do you Suntan + Do you wear Sunscreen?		**Last Skin/ Mole Check**	

MANAGE ME

Notes:
Use this area to add medical documents

Title	Document Date

MANAGE ME™
Life Management Services

Health History

Personal Health Concerns		**Hospitalizations + Dates**	
Present Medical Diagnoses		**Broken Bones**	
Past Medical Diagnoses Lifetime		**Past Reoccurring Symptoms**	
Date of Last Medical Physical		**Surgeries + Date or Age**	
Injuries Personal		**Living Will**	
Injuries Work Related		**Will (Yes/No)**	

11

MANAGE ME™
Life Management Services

Copyright © 2012 Manage Me, LMS (Life Management Systems). All rights reserved.

Health History

Current Prescriptions		**Childhood Immunizations**	
Past Prescriptions		Travel Immunizations	
Current Over the Counter Meds		Last Tetanus Shot	
Vitamins/ Minerals		Viral Infections	
Supplements		Bacterial Infections	
Adult Immunizations		Areas of recurrent Infections	

Health History

Caloric Intake/ Day Avg		**Elimination: Bowel movements X per day and consistency**	
Typical Breakfast		Elimination: Urine X per day	
Typical Lunch		Cigarette/Cigar intake	
Typical Dinner		Alcohol intake	
Typical Snacks		Recreational Drug Use	
Fluid intake (Water, coffee, tea, energy drinks, soda, juice		Cravings	

Health History

Sleep Patterns Hours in Bed		Hobbies and hours spent per week	
Sleep Patterns Hours Asleep		Current Fitness Level (Sedentary, active, athlete)	
Feel Rested upon Waking?		Practice meditation, deep breathing?	
Are pets or children in your bed?		Do you have emotional support? What do you do when feeling blue?	
Other sleep disturbance		Happiness level 0-10 (10 = Most Happy)	
Any sleep positions painful?		Seasonal affective disorder (SAD in the winter months)	

MANAGE ME™
Life Management Services

Health History

Intimacy/Sex issues?		**Oral Dental Care last check**	
Are you satisfied with your sex life?		**Tongue Check**	
STI History		**Visual Acuity + Last checkup**	
Menstrual History Age start/end		**Auditory + Last checkup**	
Do you have children? # and current age(s)		**Other**	
Do you have pets?		**Other**	

Notes:

Use this area to add medical documents

Title	Document Date

MANAGE ME™
Life Management Services

Extended Family Health History

Maternal Health Issues	Paternal Health Issues	Sibling Health Issues

Notes:

Use this area to add medical documents

MANAGE ME
Life Management Services

Screening Lab Tests

	Date/Result	Date/Result	Document Date
Blood Test Date			
Cervical/Prostate Screen			
Colorectal cancer screening			
DNA gene Testing			
Mammogram/ Testes screen			
Mental Acuteness			
MRI, CT, US etc.			
My E Health files are located:			
Screening Exam			
Skin Check			
Other			

MANAGE ME™
Life Management Services

Notes:

Use this area to add medical documents

MANAGE ME™
Life Management Services

	Date	Date	Document Date
ASSESSED CURRENT HEALTH CONCERNS			
PLAN OF ACTION			
EVALUATION/ RESULTS			
NOTES			

MANAGE ME™
Life Management Services

Notes:
Use this area to add medical documents

MANAGE ME™
Life Management Services

VITALS		Date	Date	Document Date
AREA OF NUMBNESS				
AREA OF PAIN + VAS(0-10)	0 no pain 10 extreme pain			
BLOOD PRESSURE	120/80 Normal, 140/90 Hypertension, 180/120 Hypertensive Crisis			
BMI	18.5 underweight 18.6-24.9 healthy, 25-29.9 overweight, +30 obese			
BONE DENSITY SPINE/HIP	minus-1.0 or above normal bone density. -2.5 Osteopenia. Below -2.5 osteoporosis			
FASTING BLOOD SUGAR	below 5.6 mmol/L normal 5.6 to 6.9mmol/L prediabetic. & mmol/L or > diabetic			
Heart Rate (HR)	60-100 BMP normal			
HEIGHT	ft/cm			
HRV	Measures intervals between heart beats			
NITRIC OXIDE LEVEL (LMO)	indicator of blood vessel elasticity			
OXYGEN SATS	94-99% normal, 90% needing oxygen			
PEAK FLOW METER	dependent on age see specific chart			

MANAGE ME™
Life Management Services

VITALS		Date	Date	Document Date
RESPIRATIONS	12-18 RPM normal			
Seated Height	ft/cm			
TEMP (forehead, palm, sole)	36.1 to 37.2 C normal			
WAIST Circumference	men average 18-24% women average 25-31%			
WEIGHT				
Other				

MANAGE ME™
Life Management Services

Notes:

Use this area to add medical documents

LAB RESULT MARKERS	Date		Date	Document Date
Adrenal Function				
Ferritin				
General Chemistry				
Hematology				
Hormonal Panel				
Lipids				
Liver/Kidney				
Thyroid Function				

MANAGE ME™
Life Management Services

Notes:

Use this area to add medical documents

Notes:

Use this area to add medical documents

Title	Date

Manage Me, LMS Inc.

Other publications available:

My Life Manager © Personalized Financial Records

My Health Manager © Personalized Health Records My

My Life Manager (TM)(C) APP launched 2022

www.manageme.ca

Email: info@manageme.ca

Published by Manage Me,

LMS (Life Management Systems), Inc.

MANAGE ME™
Life Management Services

www.ingramcontent.com/pod-product-compliance
Lightning Source LLC
Chambersburg PA
CBHW061137030426
42334CB00003B/71